ANTIBIOTICS AND VACCINES

Kate McArthur

NELSON
CENGAGE Learning™

Australia • Brazil • Japan • Korea • Mexico • Singapore • Spain • United Kingdom • United States

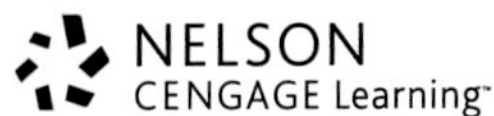

Antibiotics and Vaccines

Text: Kate McArthur
Editor: Rebecca Crisp
Design: Jennifer Warwick
Series design: James Lowe
Photo researcher: Libby Henry
Production controller: Adam Bextream
Reprint: Siew Han Ong

Acknowledgements
The author and publisher would like to acknowledge permission to reproduce material from the following sources:
akg-images: p. 16 (main); Auscape/BSIP/CHASSENET: p. 11; Corbis Australia: pp. 1, 5, cover; Elena Leong © Cengage Learning Australia: p. 15; Getty Images: pp. 12, 13, 20 (both); Photolibrary: p. 3, 4, 6, 7 (all), 10, 16 (inset), 17, 21, 22–23, back cover; Richard Morden © Cengage Learning Australia: pp. 8–9, 18–19.

Every effort has been made to trace and acknowledge copyright. However, if any infringement has occurred the publishers tender their apologies and invite the copyright holders to contact them.

Fast Forward Independent Texts Level 22

For product information and technology assistance,
in Australia call 1300 790 853;
in New Zealand call 0508 635 766

For permission to use material from this text or product,
please email **aust.permissions@cengage.com**

ISBN 978 0 17 017993 5
ISBN 978 0 17 017899 0 (set)

Cengage Learning Australia
Level 7, 80 Dorcas Street
South Melbourne, Victoria Australia 3205

Cengage Learning New Zealand
Unit 4B Rosedale Office Park
331 Rosedale Road, Albany, North Shore NZ 0632

For learning solutions, visit **cengage.com.au**

Printed in Australia by Ligare Pty Ltd
2 3 4 5 6 7 22 21 20 29

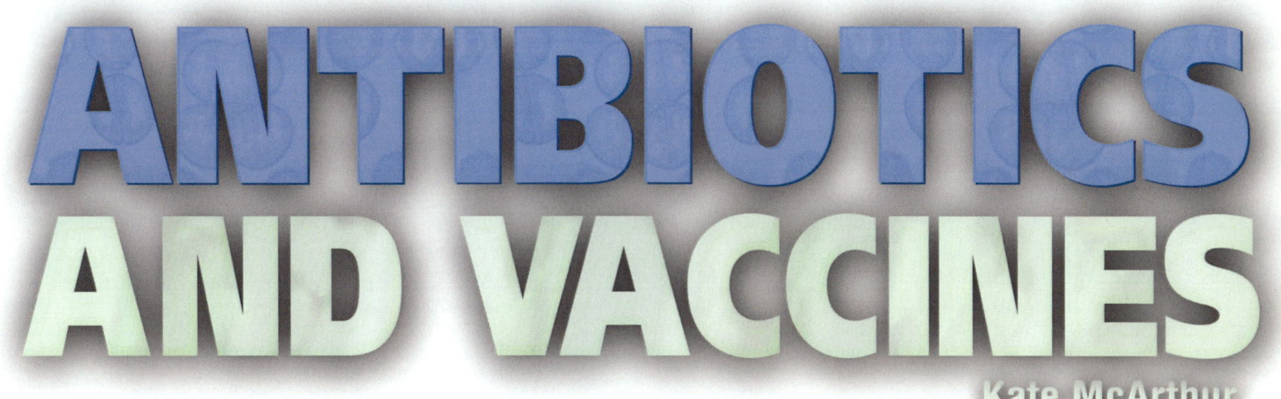

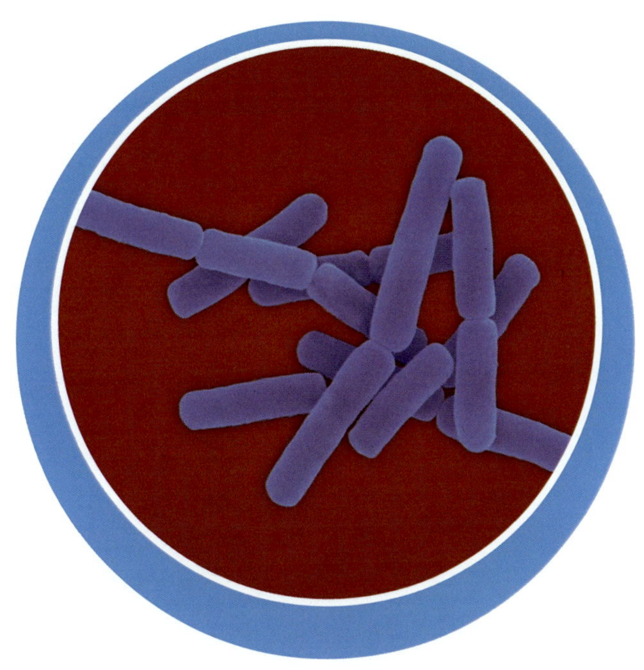

Contents

Chapter 1 Fighting Infection and Disease 4
Chapter 2 Bacteria and Antibiotics 6
Chapter 3 Viruses and Vaccines 10
Chapter 4 The History of Antibiotics and Vaccines 12
Chapter 5 The Dangers of Overusing Antibiotics 18
Chapter 6 The Future of Antibiotics and Vaccines 22
Glossary and Index 24

CHAPTER 1

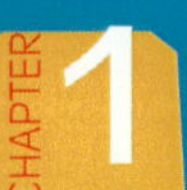

Fighting Infection and Disease

Antibiotics and vaccines are used to **cure** and prevent sickness. They are two of the most important medical discoveries ever made.

There are two main types of germs that can cause infection and disease: **bacteria** and **viruses**.

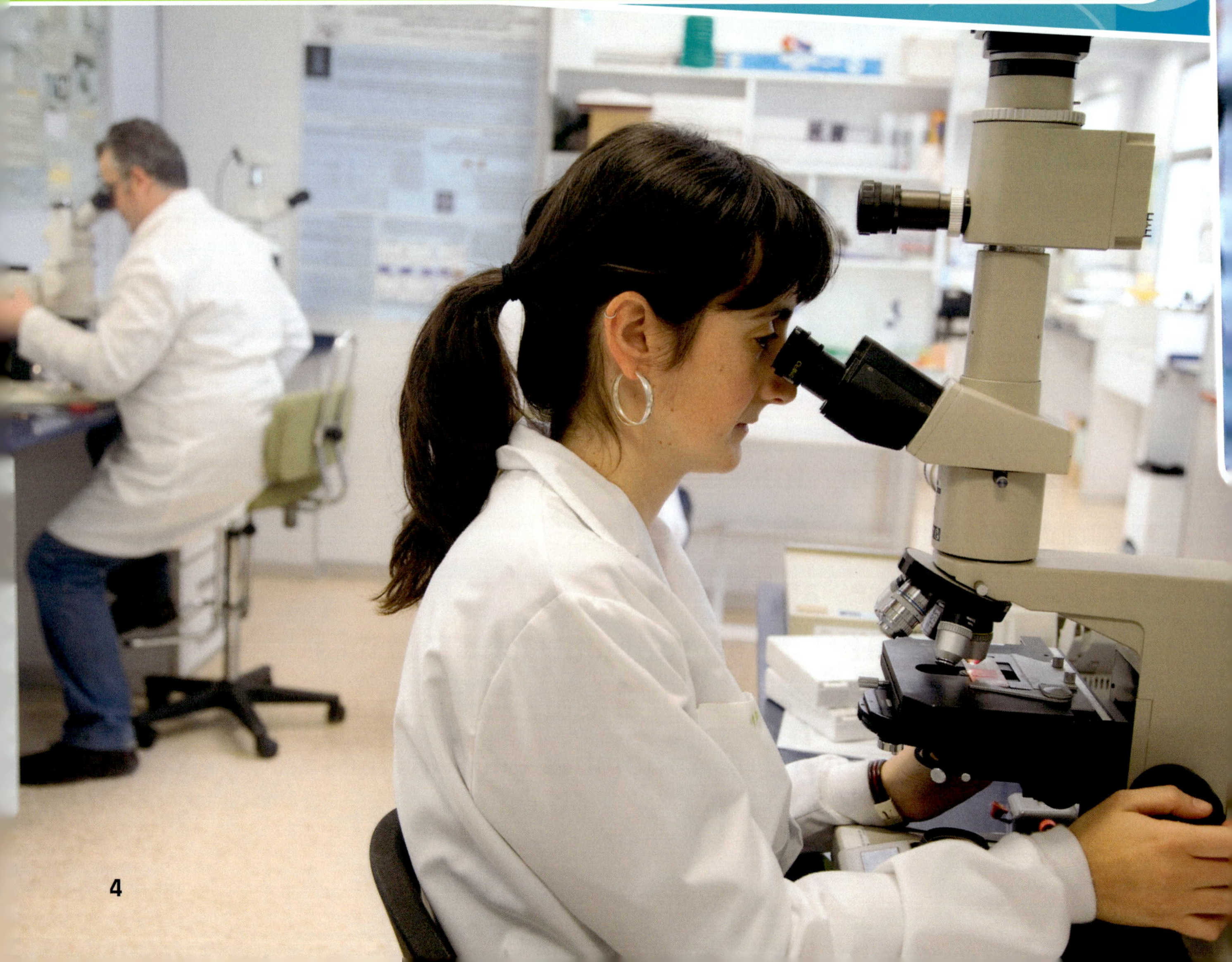

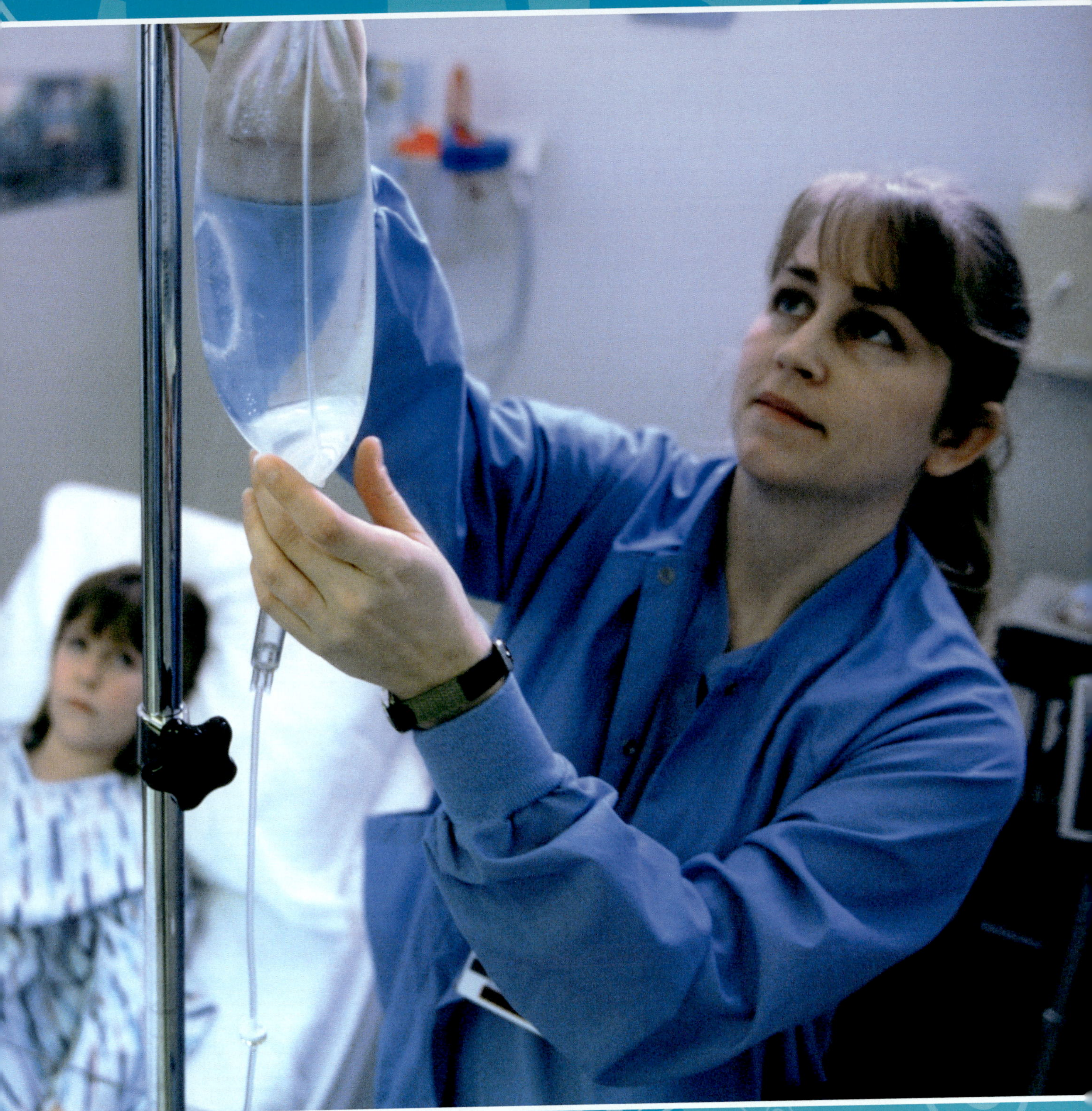

Doctors use antibiotics to cure sickness
when bacteria infect the body.
Diseases caused by viruses cannot usually
be cured by antibiotics,
but sometimes they can be prevented by vaccines.

CHAPTER 2

Bacteria and Antibiotics

Bacteria are tiny living things that can only be seen under a microscope.

Bacteria can grow quickly and can survive almost anywhere on Earth. They can live in people's bodies, in water, in the ground and on things that people touch.

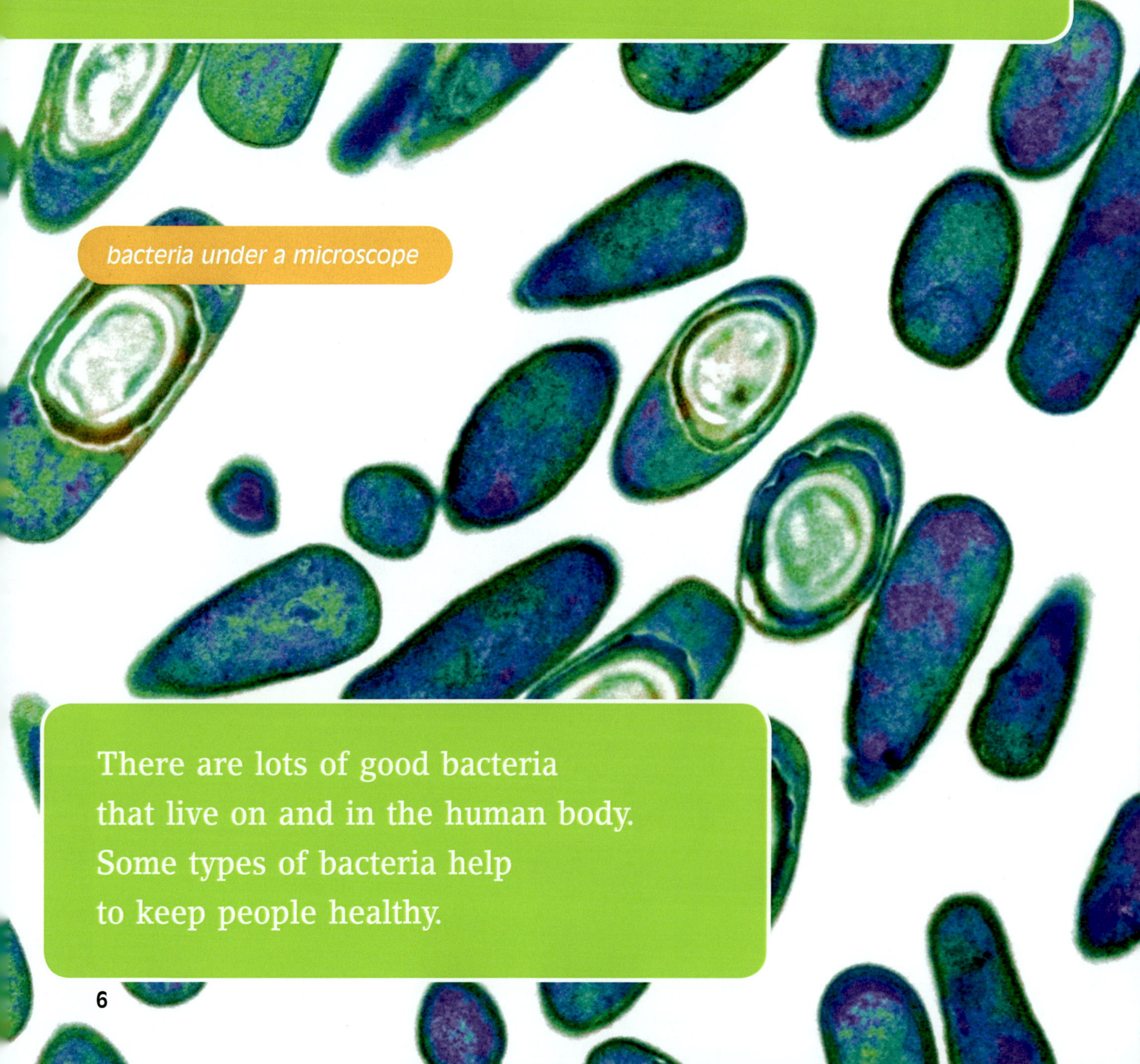

bacteria under a microscope

There are lots of good bacteria that live on and in the human body. Some types of bacteria help to keep people healthy.

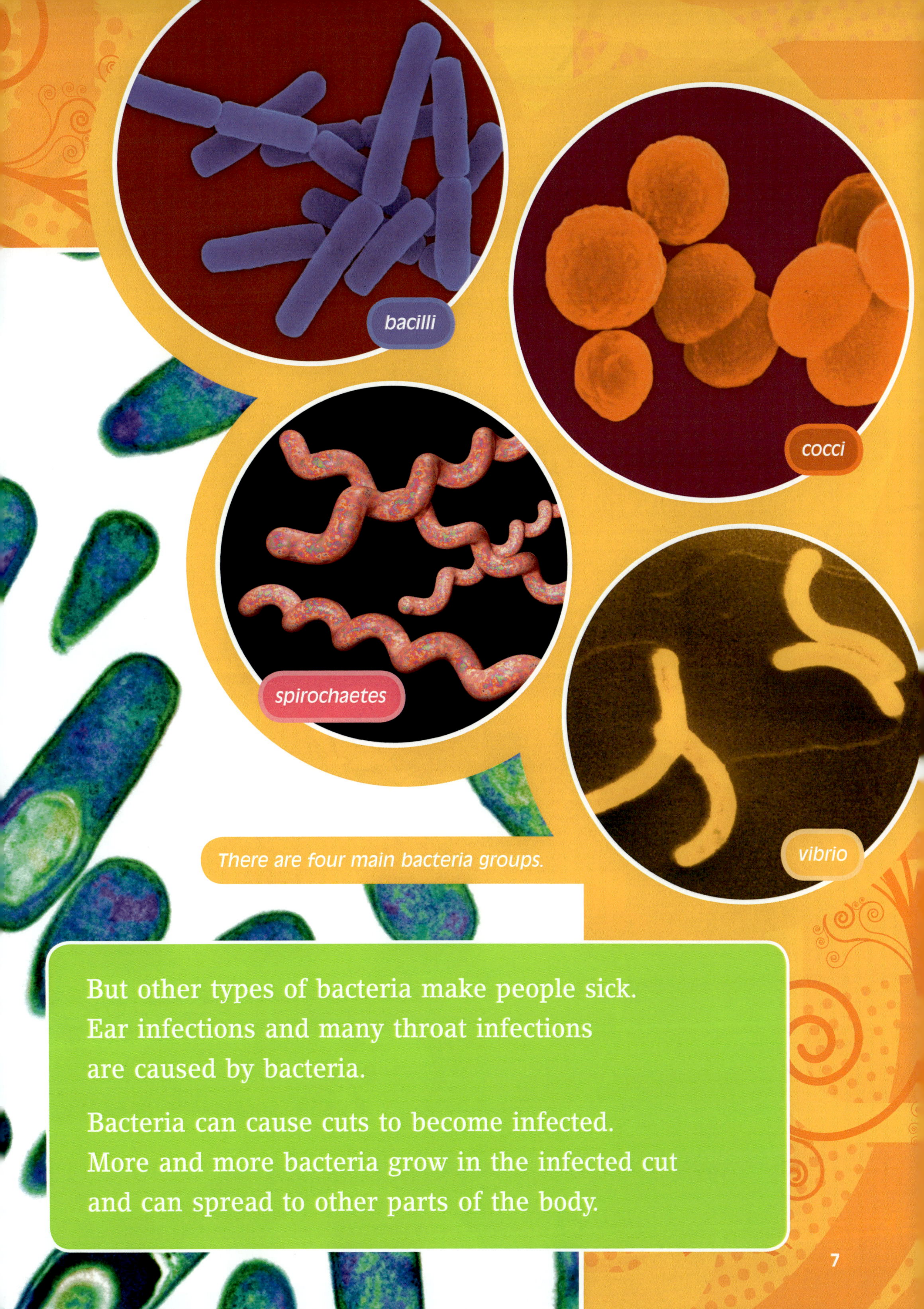

There are four main bacteria groups.

But other types of bacteria make people sick. Ear infections and many throat infections are caused by bacteria.

Bacteria can cause cuts to become infected. More and more bacteria grow in the infected cut and can spread to other parts of the body.

The human body has an immune system.
Usually when people get sick,
the immune system fights the sickness
and people get better without antibiotics.
The immune system gets stronger
as it fights the bacteria.

But sometimes the body's immune system needs help.
Antibiotics are chemicals
that help the body win the fight by killing bacteria
or stopping them from growing.
Once the bacteria have been killed,
the body's immune system cleans up
all the dead bacteria.

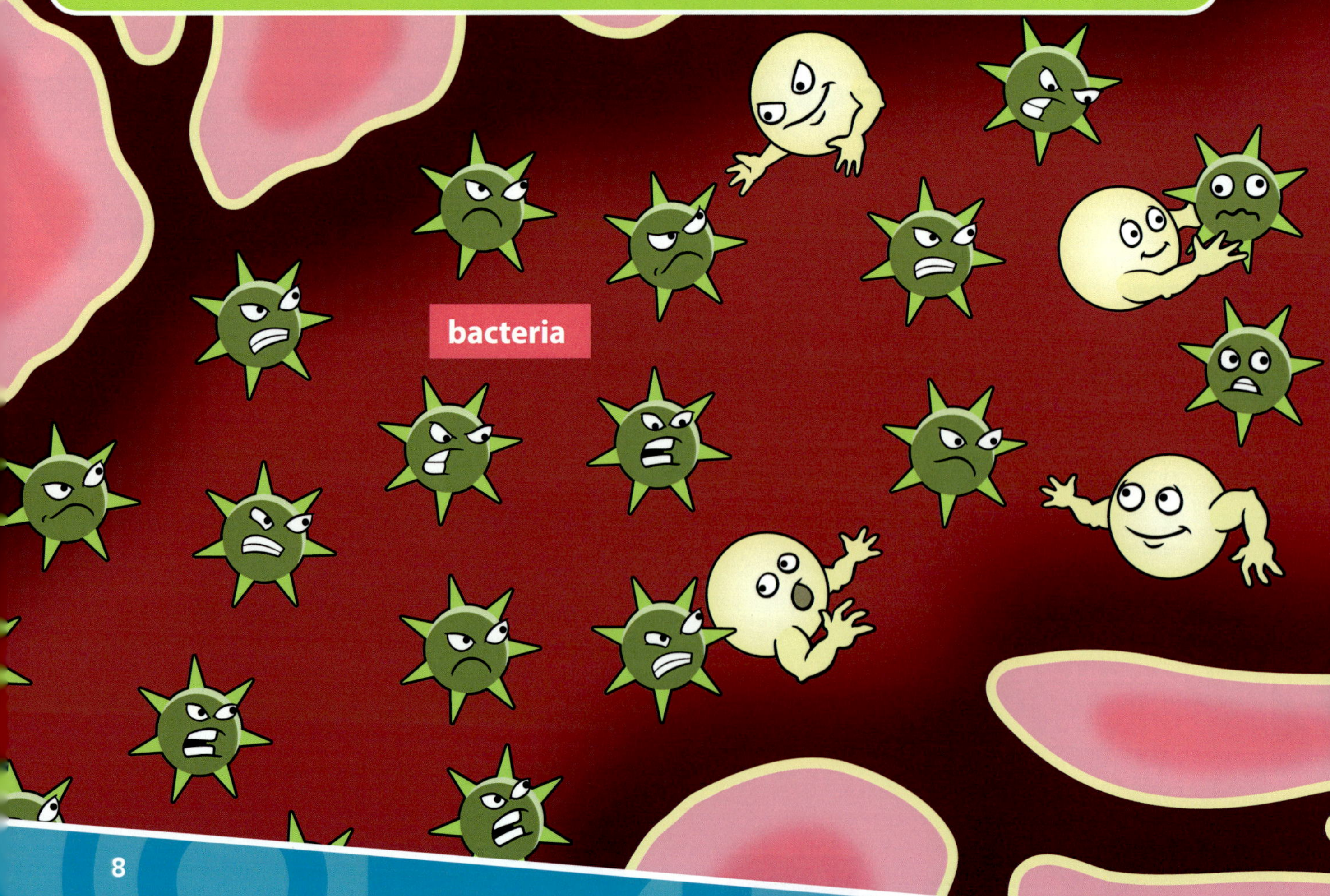

The immune system is like an army that defends the body against invasion by harmful bacteria. When bacteria enter the body, the immune system makes **antibodies**, which act like soldiers to search out and destroy the harmful bacteria. Antibiotics help antibodies in the fight against harmful bacteria.

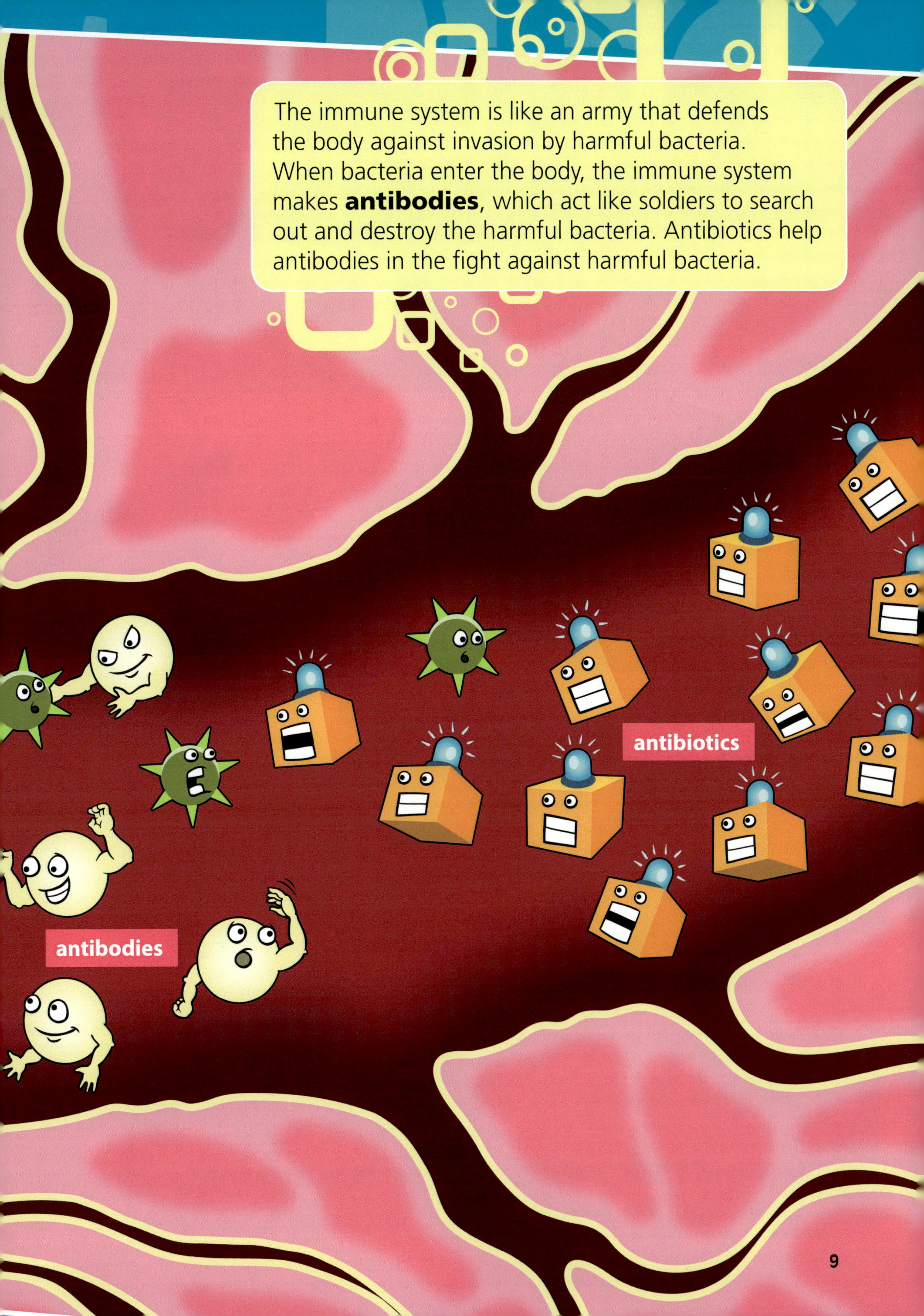

CHAPTER 3

Viruses and Vaccines

Viruses are different from bacteria.
Viruses depend on other living **cells** to survive,
and they stay in the body
unless the body can defend itself.

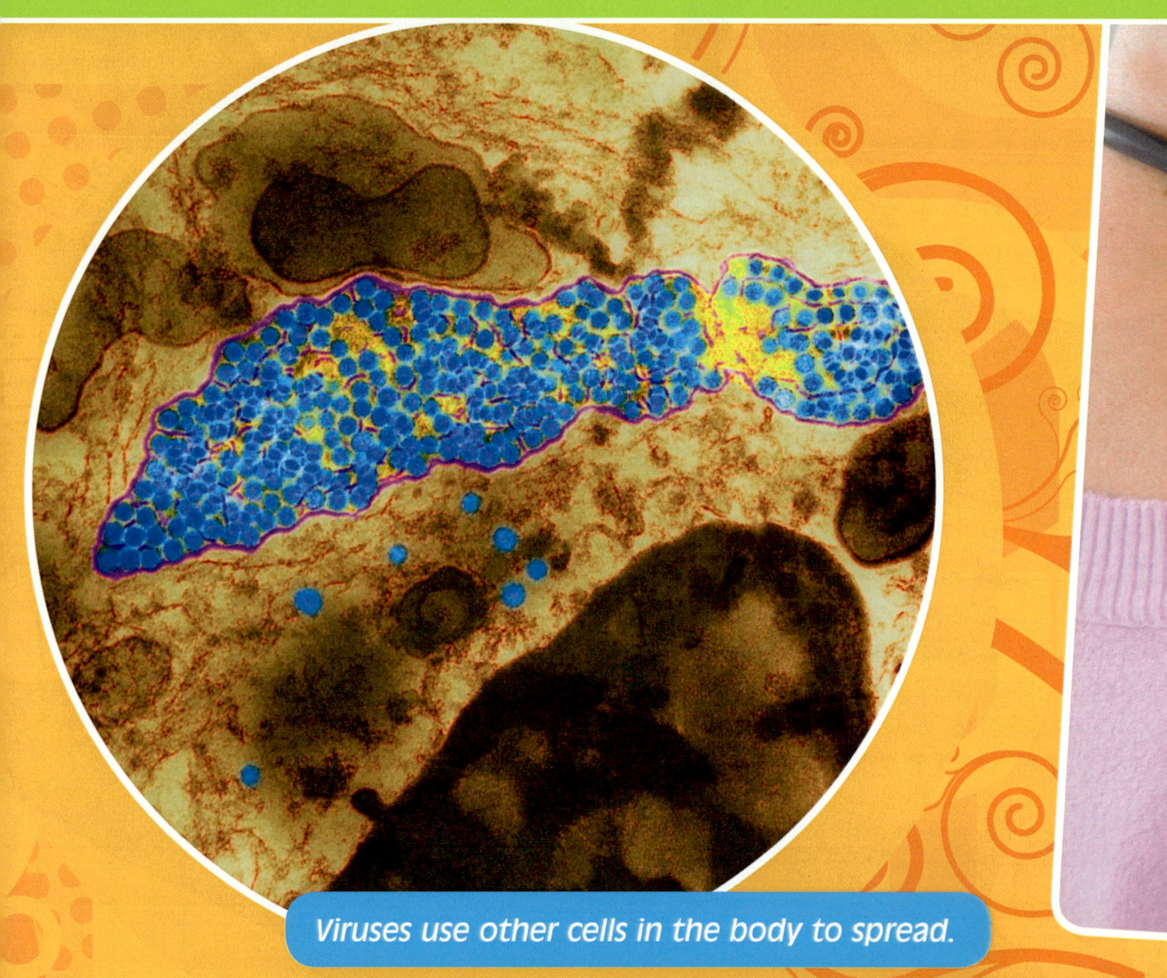

Viruses use other cells in the body to spread.

Usually, the body develops ways of fighting the virus.
It learns how to beat the virus
so it cannot ever invade the body again.
This is called developing immunity.

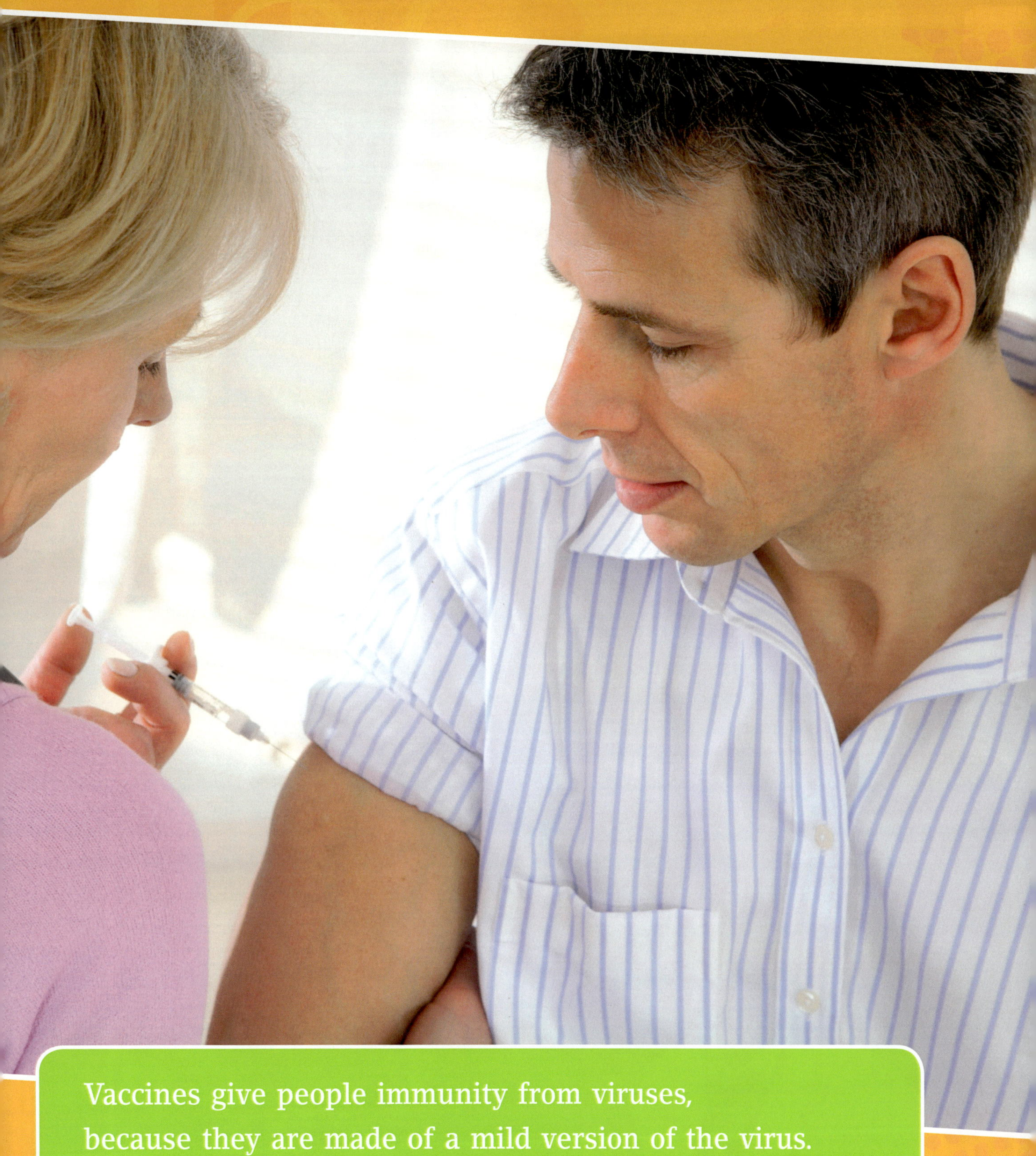

Vaccines give people immunity from viruses, because they are made of a mild version of the virus. Vaccines make the body's immune system stronger by helping it develop antibodies that will attack the virus when it enters the body and stop the virus from causing sickness.

CHAPTER 4

The History of Antibiotics and Vaccines

Alexander Fleming discovered the world's first antibiotic by chance in 1928. He called it penicillin.

More research carried out by other scientists meant that by 1945, the USA was making enough penicillin to give 34 million **doses** every day. By 1972, people were living for up to eight years longer because of antibiotics.

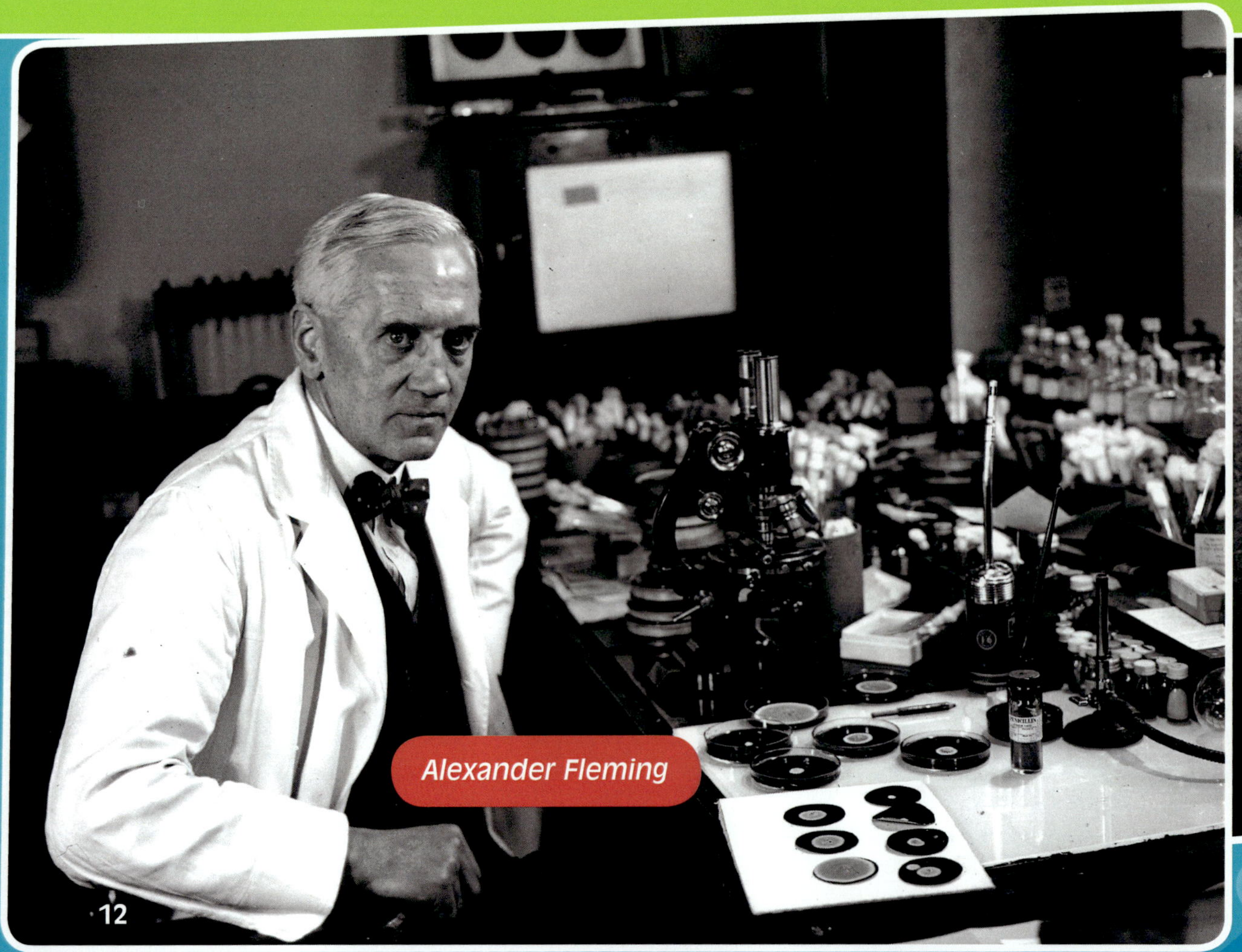

Alexander Fleming

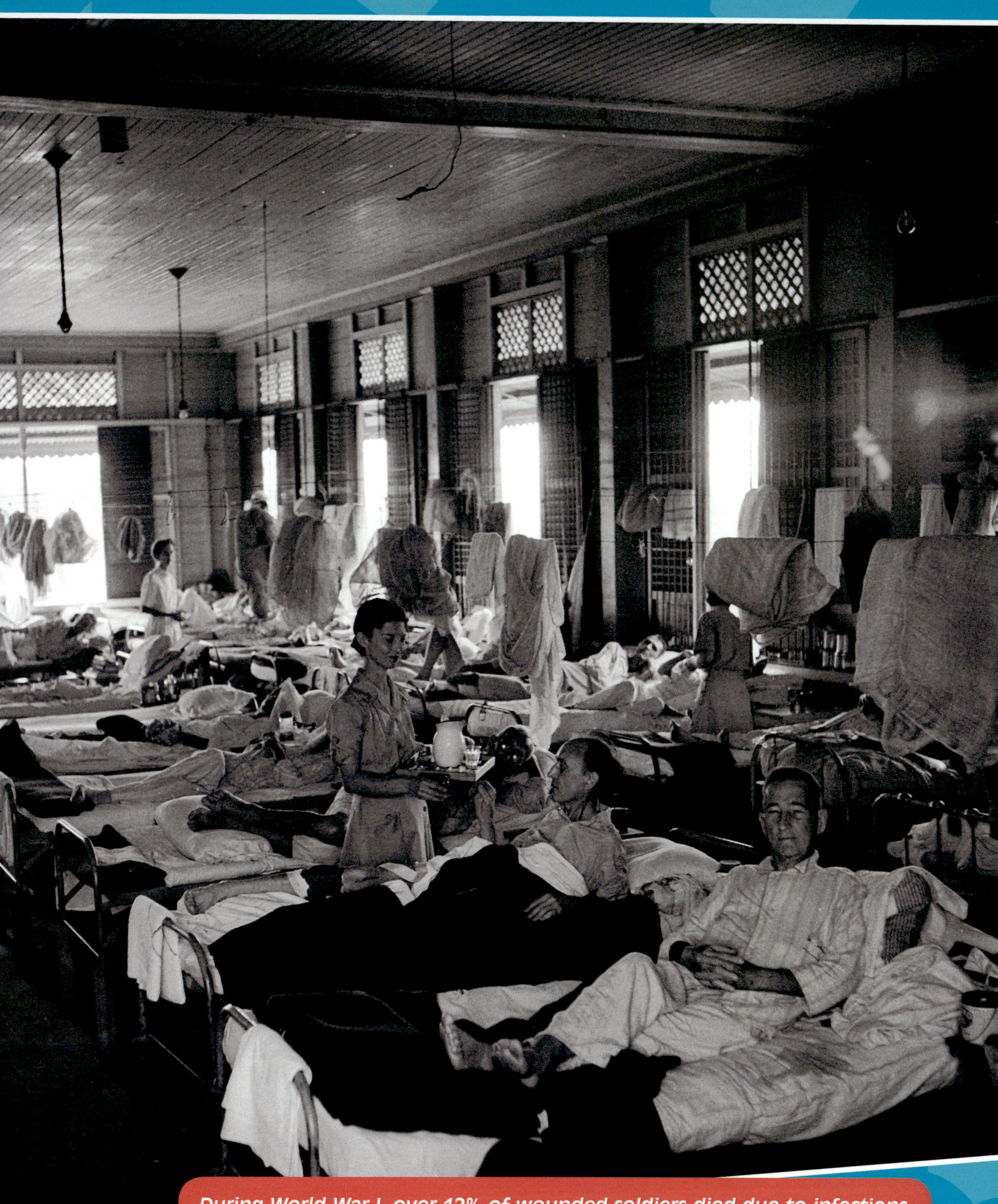

During World War I, over 12% of wounded soldiers died due to infections. During World War II, this number was almost zero because of antibiotics.

Vaccines have been used
for much longer than antibiotics.

Even before people knew much
about the causes of disease,
they noticed that if a disease didn't kill them,
they would often be immune from catching it
a second time.

In the 1700s,
Chinese doctors used this observation
to try to make people immune to **smallpox**.

Chinese Methods for Creating Immunity to Smallpox

1. Take pus from the blisters of an infected person and inject it into non-infected people.
2. Remove scabs from smallpox blisters, grind them into a powder and give the powder to non-infected people to breathe in.
3. Inject this same powder into non-infected people.

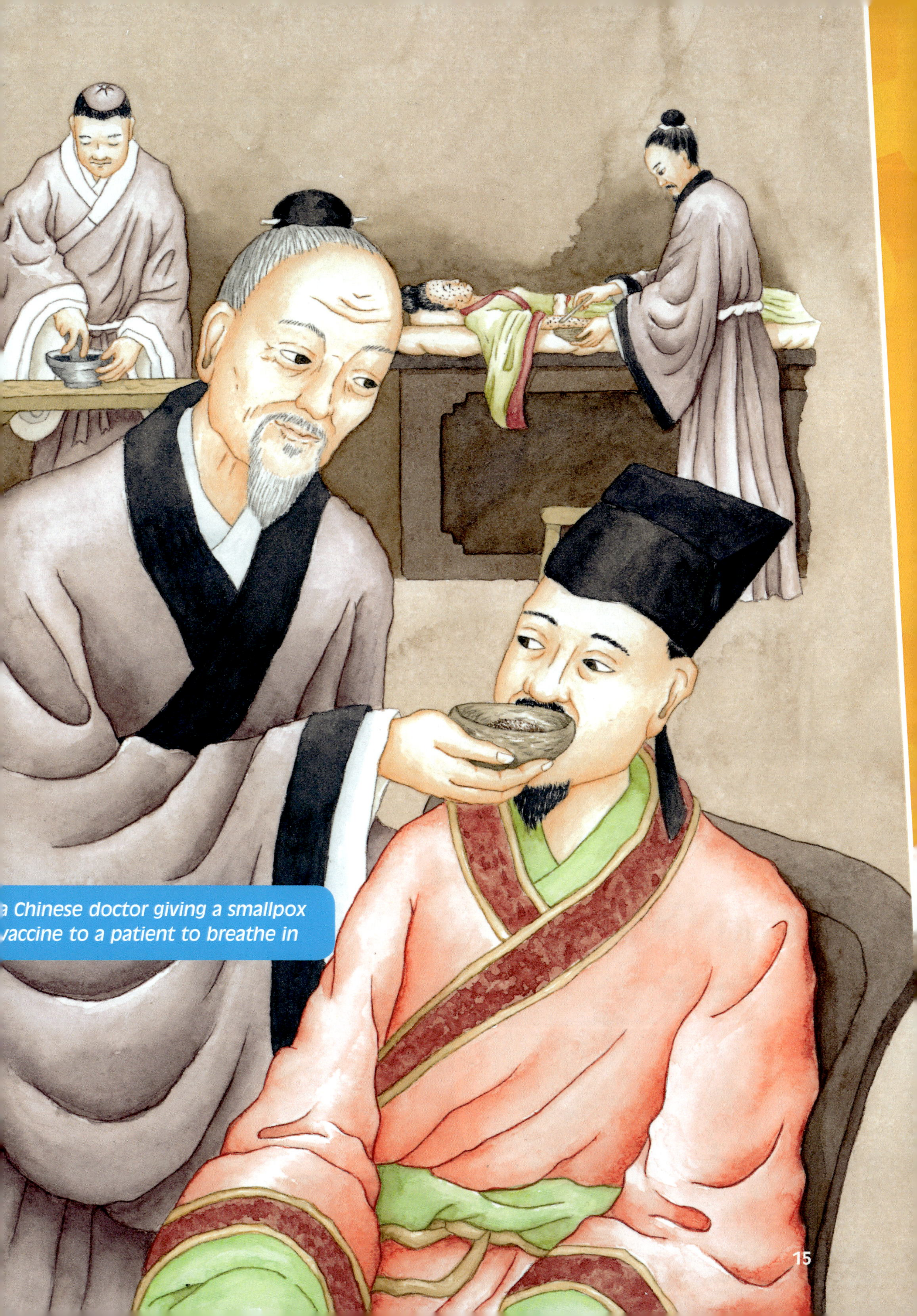

a Chinese doctor giving a smallpox vaccine to a patient to breathe in

In the 1790s, Edward Jenner made a vaccine for smallpox.
Doctors around the world began to **immunise** people against the disease, saving thousands of lives.

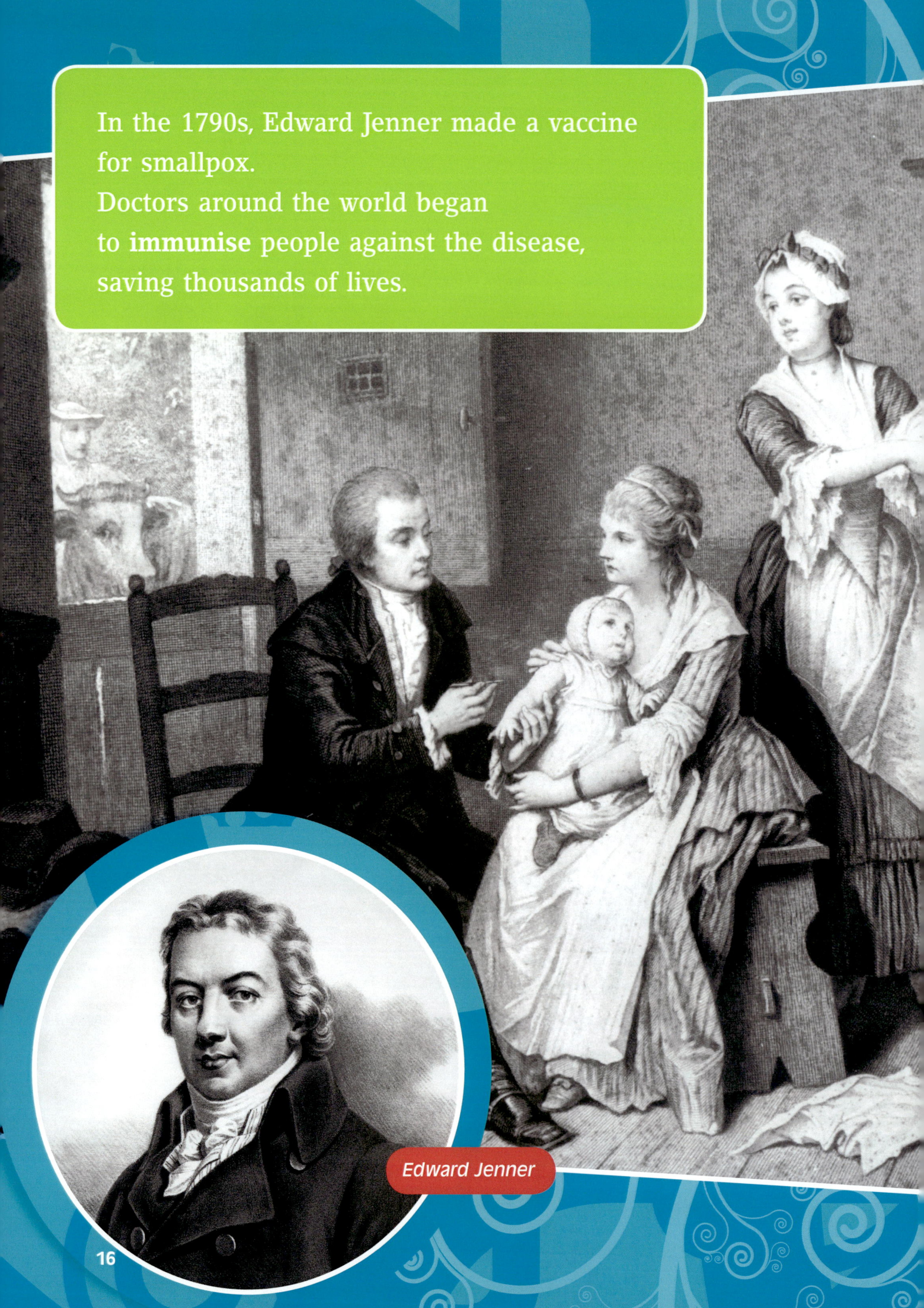

Edward Jenner

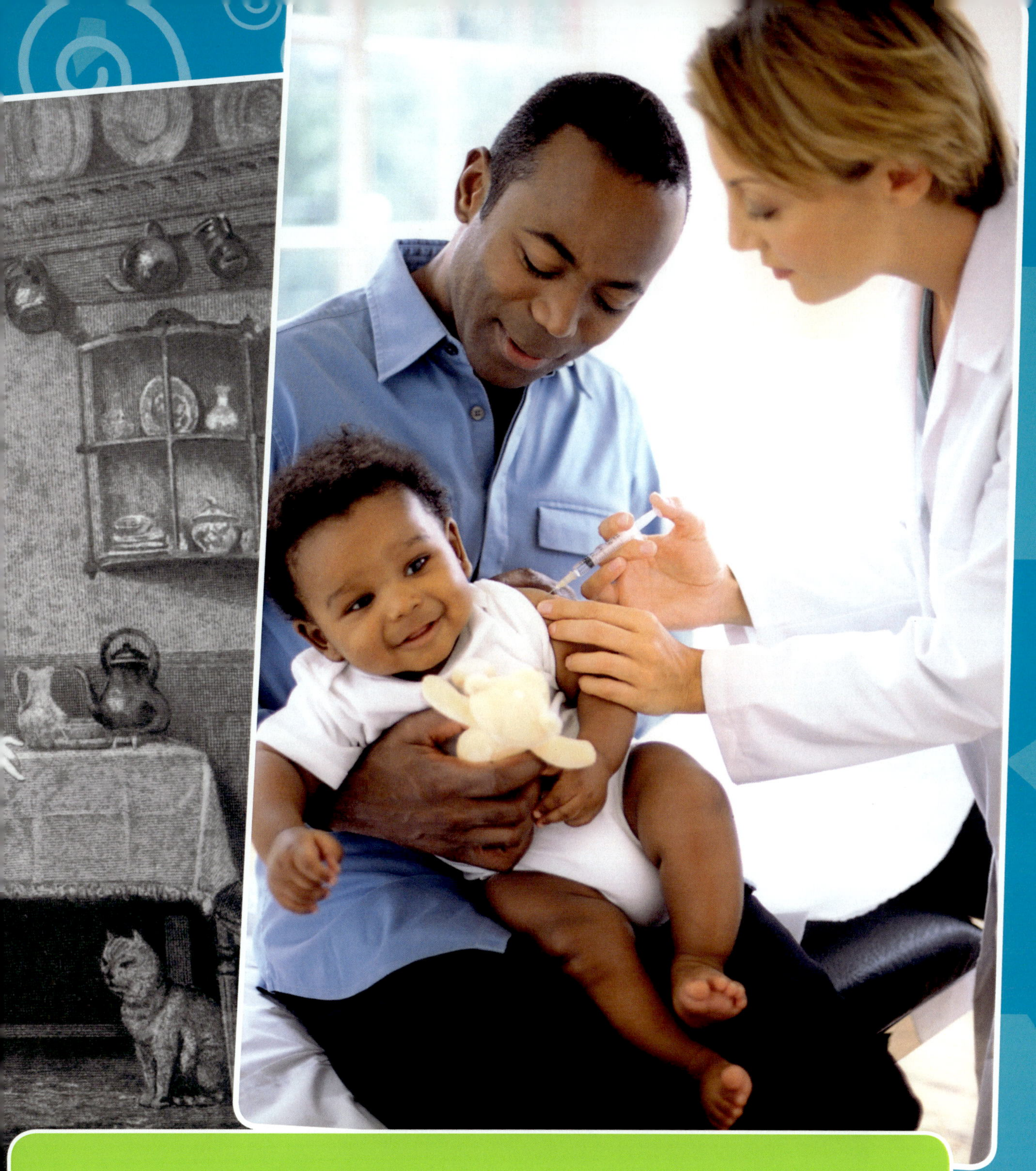

Today, vaccines are so common that most children receive a number of them before they turn one year old.

Many diseases that once killed hundreds of thousands of people have almost disappeared because of vaccines.

The Dangers of Overusing Antibiotics

Antibiotics can kill good bacteria inside the body, so sometimes they do more harm than good.

When antibiotics are used too much, curing some diseases becomes difficult. Bacteria sometimes learn how to fight against antibiotics, so the antibiotics don't work as well. These bacteria have become **resistant** to antibiotics.

There are different reasons why bacteria become resistant to antibiotics.

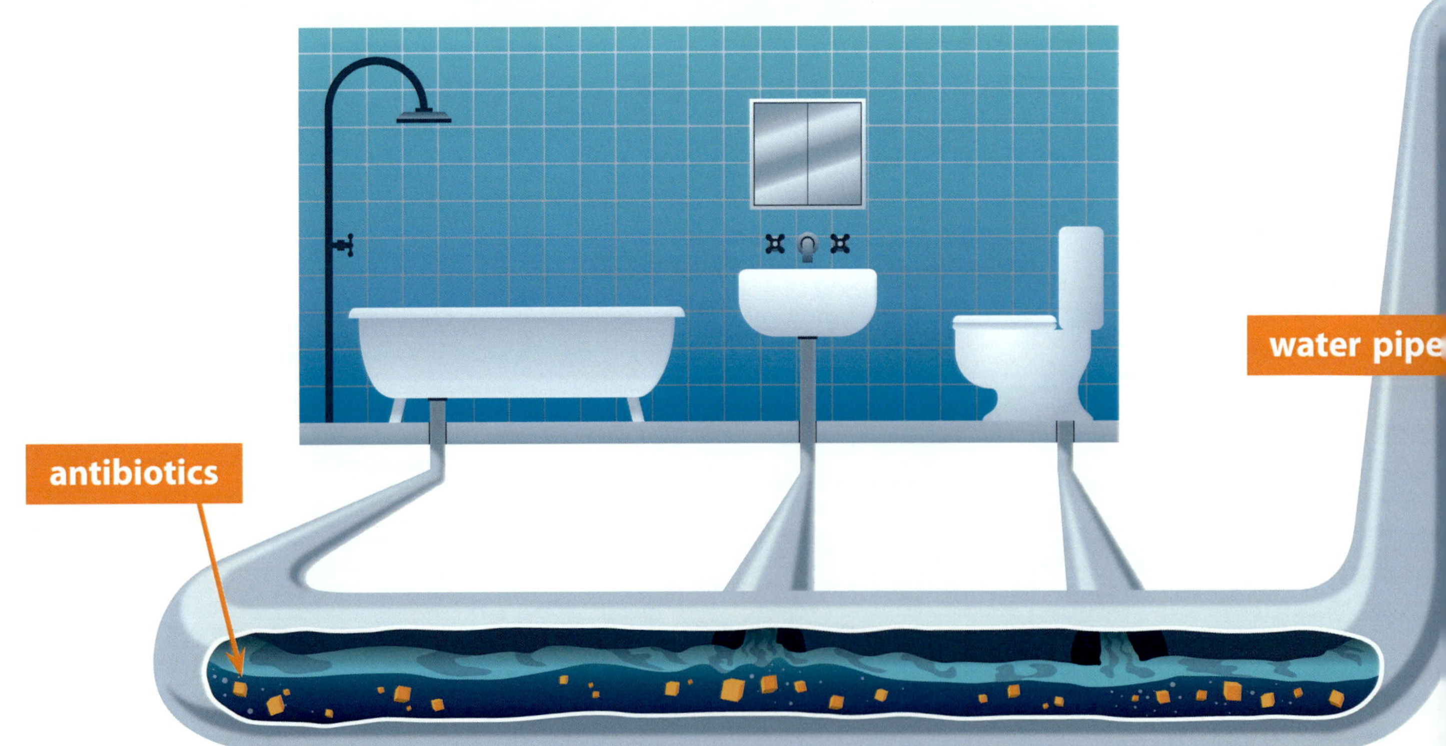

Antibiotics come out of people's bodies when they wash themselves or use the toilet.

When a lot of antibiotics enter the environment, the bacteria in the environment change. Huge amounts of antibiotics go into the environment every day. Many antibiotics come out of people's bodies as waste and end up in the water system.

Lots of antibiotics enter the water system through people's homes and end up in the environment.

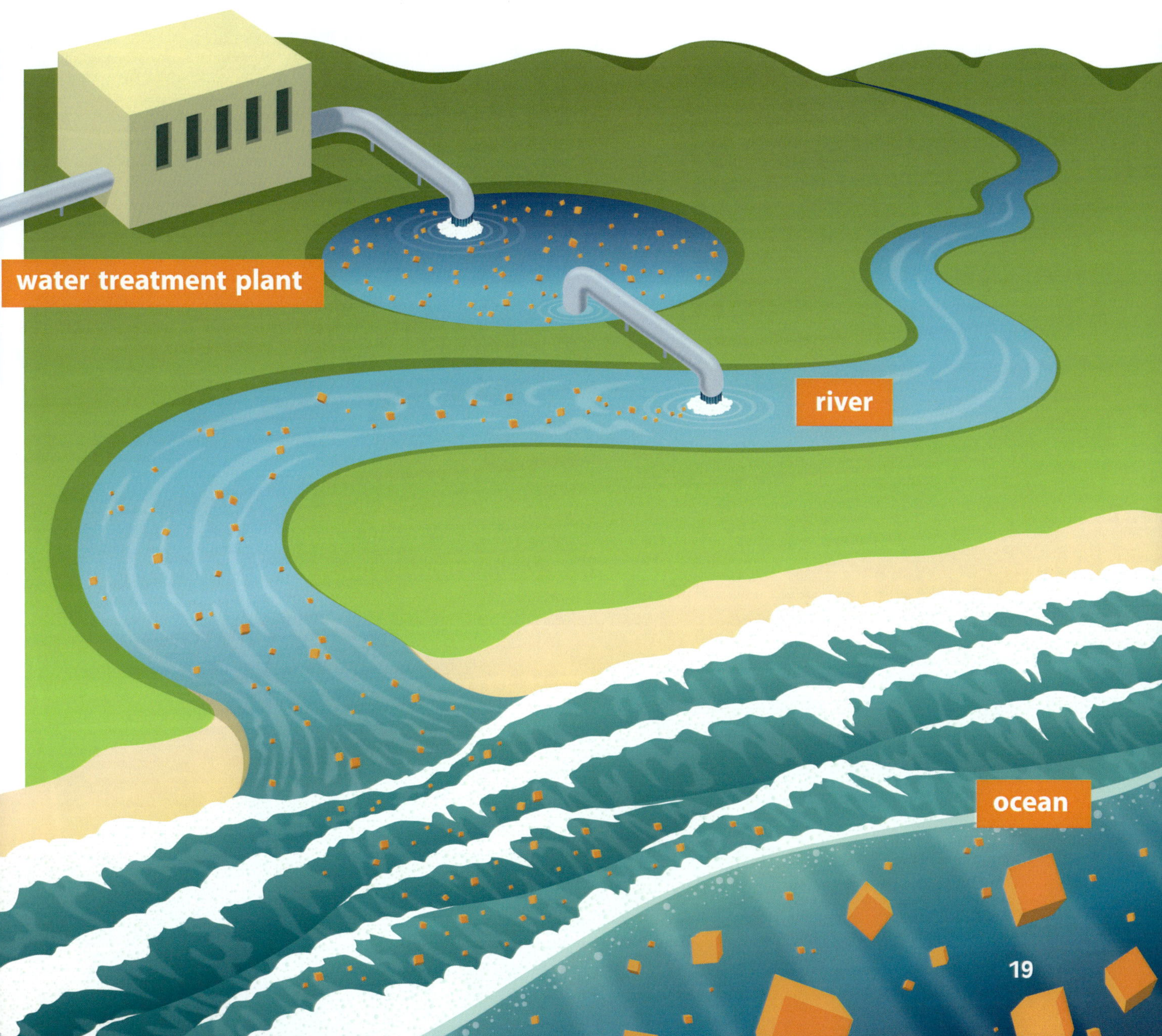

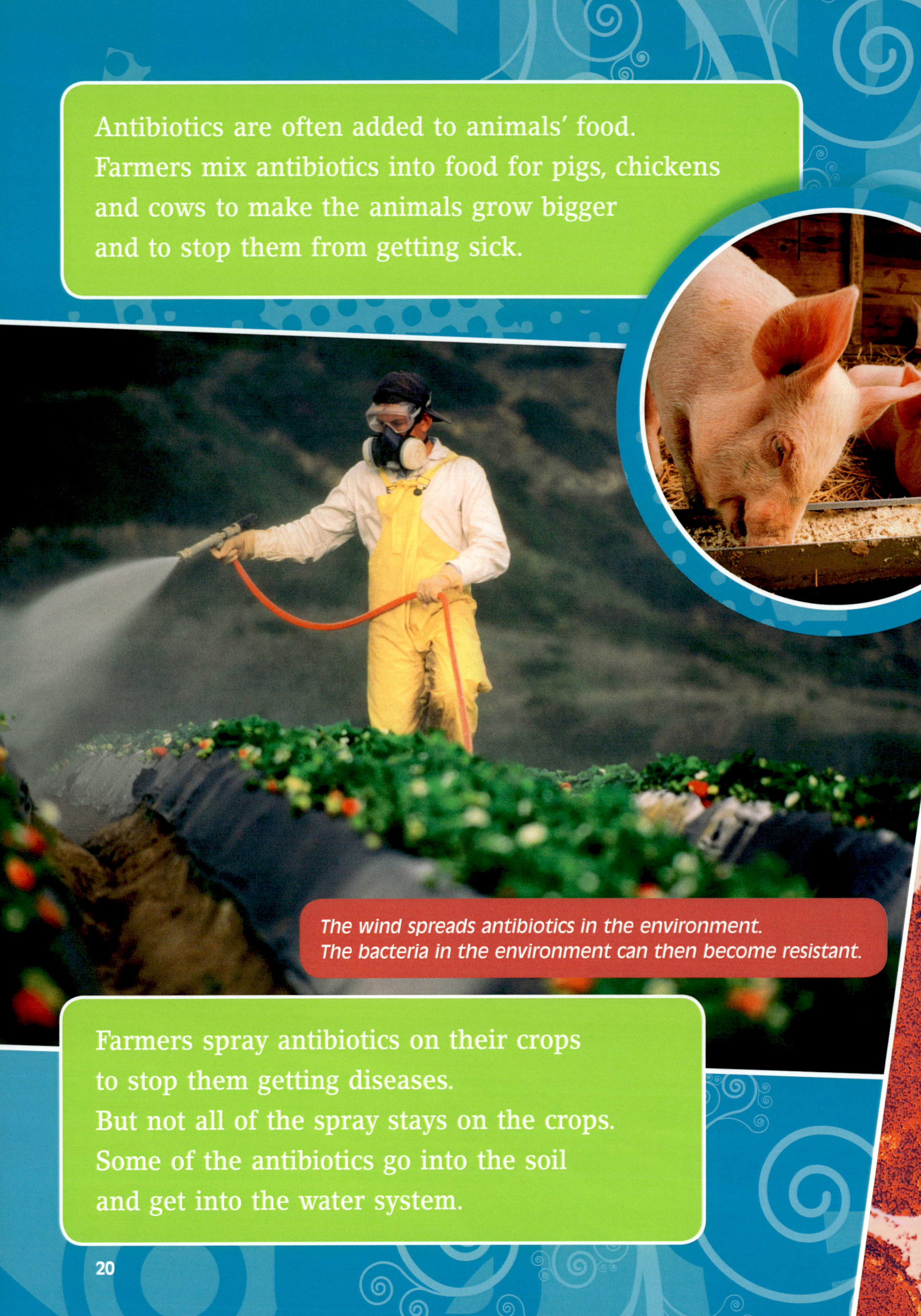

Antibiotics are often added to animals' food. Farmers mix antibiotics into food for pigs, chickens and cows to make the animals grow bigger and to stop them from getting sick.

The wind spreads antibiotics in the environment. The bacteria in the environment can then become resistant.

Farmers spray antibiotics on their crops to stop them getting diseases. But not all of the spray stays on the crops. Some of the antibiotics go into the soil and get into the water system.

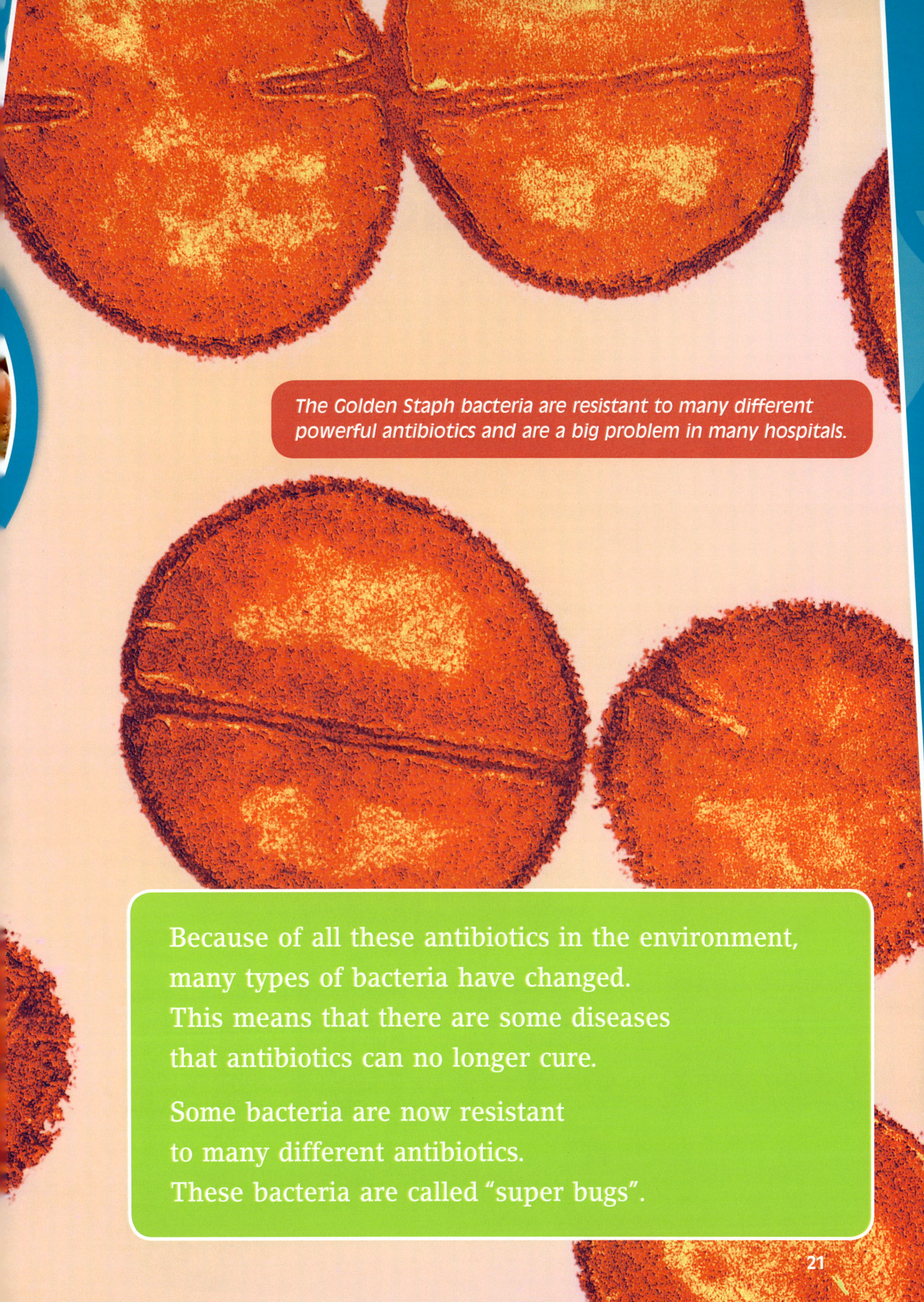

The Golden Staph bacteria are resistant to many different powerful antibiotics and are a big problem in many hospitals.

Because of all these antibiotics in the environment, many types of bacteria have changed. This means that there are some diseases that antibiotics can no longer cure.

Some bacteria are now resistant to many different antibiotics. These bacteria are called “super bugs”.

CHAPTER 6

The Future of Antibiotics and Vaccines

Since antibiotics and vaccines were first discovered, they have been used to cure and prevent much pain, disease and suffering.
They have helped people to live longer, and have saved millions of lives all around the world.

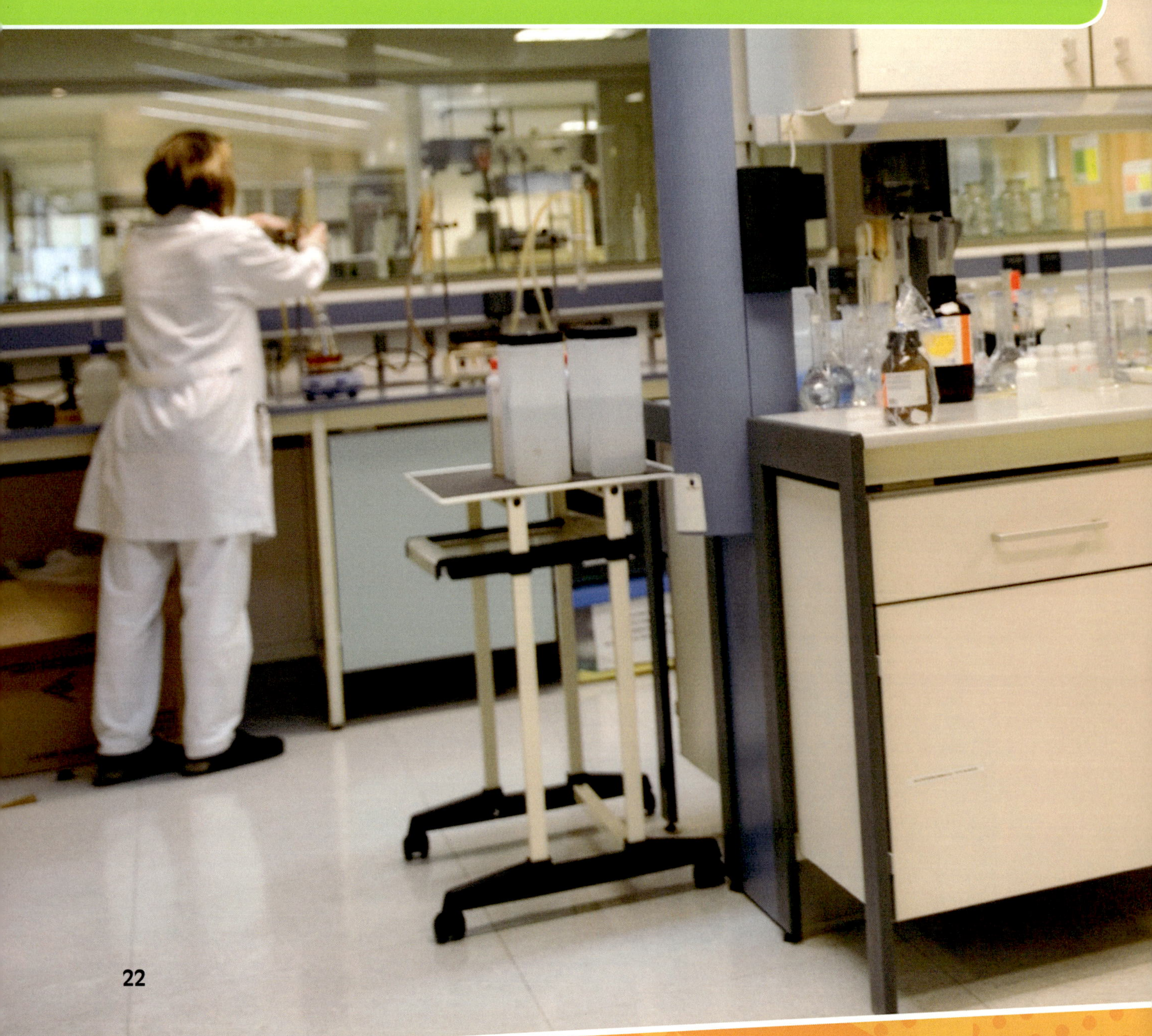

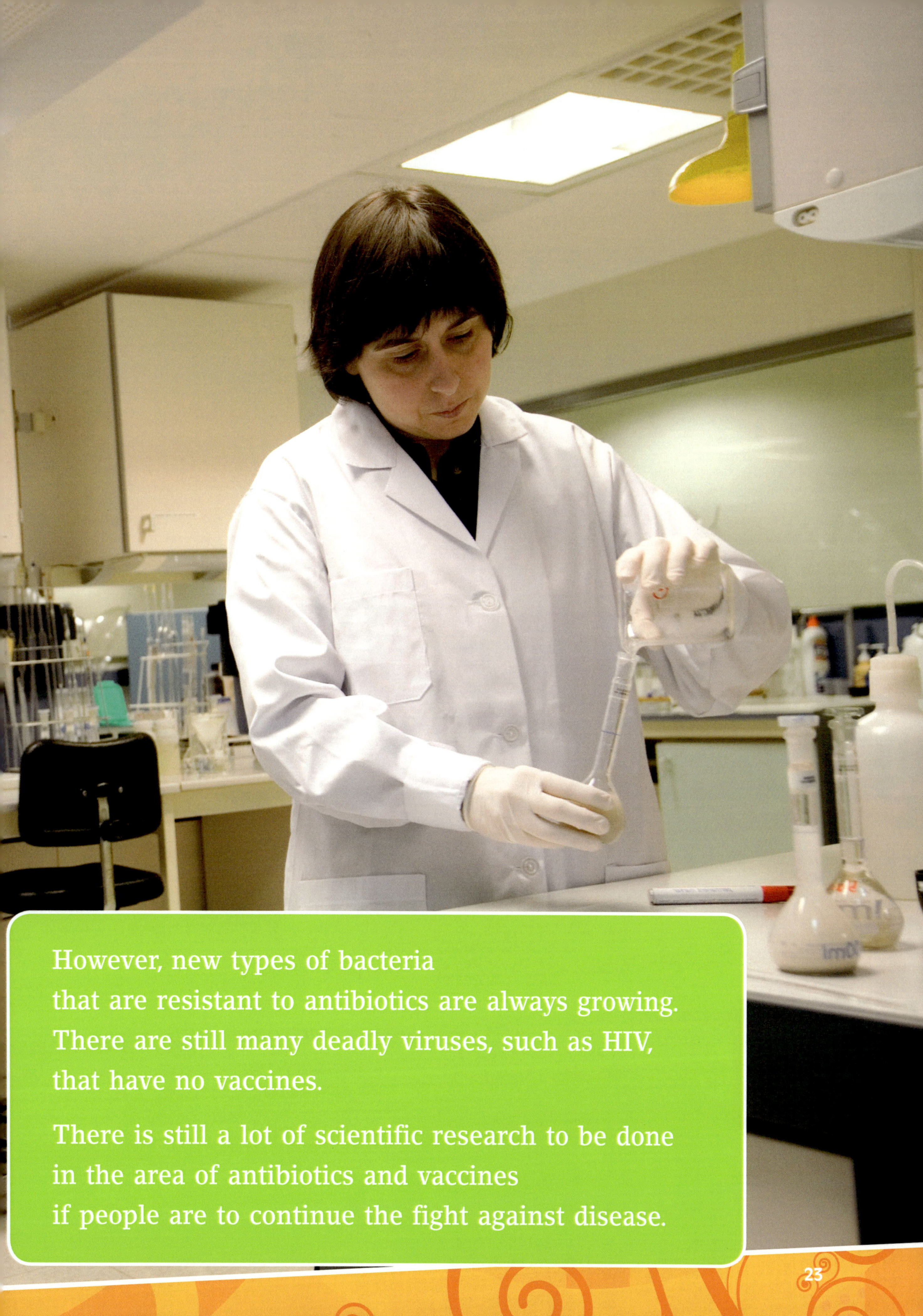

However, new types of bacteria
that are resistant to antibiotics are always growing.
There are still many deadly viruses, such as HIV,
that have no vaccines.

There is still a lot of scientific research to be done
in the area of antibiotics and vaccines
if people are to continue the fight against disease.

Glossary

antibodies substances produced by the body as a natural defence against disease

bacteria tiny single-cell organisms that can only be seen under a powerful microscope

cells tiny building blocks of life

cure to get rid of a sickness

doses amounts of medicine to be taken at one time

immunise to protect against a disease

resistant able to fight against something

smallpox a disease that causes fever and a rash of red lumps, or "pocks" on the skin

viruses tiny germs that can only reproduce inside the cells of something living

Index

bacteria 4–8, 10, 18–19, 21, 23

cells 10

Chinese 14

disease 4–5, 14, 16–18, 20–23

farmers 20

Fleming, Alexander 12

germs 4

immune system 8, 11

Jenner, Edward 16

penicillin 12

smallpox 14, 16

super bugs 21

viruses 4–5, 10–11, 23